INTRODUCTION

Welcome to "Metabolic Confusion Made Simple: A Step-by-Step Guide to Effortless Weight Loss." If you've ever felt frustrated by the ups and downs of traditional diets, you're not alone. The journey to sustainable weight loss can be a confusing maze of conflicting information and one-size-fits-all approaches.

But what if there was a revolutionary way to tap into your body's innate ability to burn fat efficiently without the stress of restrictive diets or exhaustive workouts? Enter the world of Metabolic Confusion – a groundbreaking concept that transforms weight loss from a struggle into a seamless, empowering journey.

In the following pages, we'll demystify the science behind metabolic confusion and provide you with a clear, actionable roadmap to harness its power for your transformation. This isn't just another diet book; it's a guide to understanding and optimizing your body's metabolism in a natural, sustainable, and effortless way.

What Awaits You:

1.   The Basics of Metabolism: We'll unravel metabolism's

mysteries, breaking down complex concepts into easy-to-understand terms. Understanding your body's inner workings is the first step toward unlocking its full potential.

2. The Science Behind Metabolic Confusion: Delve into the research and studies that form the foundation of the Metabolic Confusion approach. Learn how simple shifts in your eating patterns can kickstart your metabolism, making weight loss a natural byproduct of your lifestyle.

3. Practical Principles: Discover the core principles of the Metabolic Confusion Diet. From caloric cycling to strategic macronutrient adjustments, we'll guide you through creating a personalized plan that fits seamlessly into your life.

4. Your Customized Plan: No two bodies are the same, and neither should your weight loss approach. We'll walk you through assessing your unique metabolic needs and crafting a plan that aligns with your goals, preferences, and lifestyle.

5. Real Stories, Real Results: Hear the inspiring stories of individuals who have embraced the Metabolic Confusion lifestyle and witnessed transformative results. Their experiences will motivate and guide you on your journey.

6. Integration with Exercise: Understand how to synergize the power of Metabolic Confusion with your workout routine. Whether you're a fitness enthusiast or just starting, we'll explore how to optimize your exercise for maximum metabolic impact.

7. Beyond the Scale: This isn't just about shedding pounds; it's about achieving holistic well-being. Explore

down nutrients from food into simpler forms, such as the breakdown of carbohydrates into glucose or fats into fatty acids and glycerol.

Key Points About Metabolism:

• Energy Production: One crucial aspect of metabolism is the production of energy. The energy derived from the breakdown of nutrients is often stored as adenosine triphosphate (ATP), which serves as a universal energy currency for cellular processes.

• Enzymes: Metabolic reactions are facilitated by enzymes, which act as catalysts, speeding up the rate of chemical reactions without being consumed.

• Nutrient Processing: Metabolism processes different types of nutrients, including carbohydrates, fats, proteins, and vitamins, to meet the energy and structural needs of the body.

• Regulation: Metabolic processes are tightly regulated to maintain a balance and respond to the body's changing needs. Hormones, produced by endocrine glands, play a crucial role in regulating metabolic activities.

• Cellular Respiration: In eukaryotic cells, an essential process involved in metabolism is cellular respiration, where cells use oxygen to convert glucose into ATP, releasing carbon dioxide and water as byproducts.

Various factors, including genetics, age, sex, body composition, and physical activity, influence metabolism. Understanding metabolism is essential for comprehending how the body processes nutrients, maintains energy balance, and manages various physiological functions.

How Metabolism Affects Weight Management

Metabolism plays a crucial role in weight management, influencing how the body uses and stores energy from food. Understanding how metabolism affects weight management is critical in developing effective weight loss, weight maintenance, or muscle gain strategies. It emphasizes the importance of a balanced diet, regular physical activity, and lifestyle factors in achieving and sustaining a healthy weight. Additionally, factors promoting metabolic health, such as adequate sleep, stress management, and hydration, contribute to overall well-being and influence weight management outcomes.

Several factors contribute to the relationship between metabolism and weight:

1. Basal Metabolic Rate (BMR): BMR represents the calories needed to maintain basic physiological functions at rest, such as breathing, circulation, and maintaining body temperature. A higher BMR means the body burns more calories at rest, contributing to weight loss if caloric intake is controlled.

2. Caloric Expenditure: Metabolism accounts for the majority of the calories burned daily. Physical activity, including exercise and daily activities, contributes to total caloric expenditure. A higher metabolism can result in more efficient calorie burning during rest and physical activity.

3. Caloric Intake: The calories consumed through food and beverages must be balanced with the calories expended

through metabolism and physical activity. If caloric intake exceeds expenditure, the excess energy is stored as fat, leading to weight gain. Conversely, a caloric deficit, where expenditure exceeds intake, can result in weight loss.

4. Metabolic Rate Variability: People's metabolic rates are influenced by age, genetics, body composition, and hormonal levels. Some individuals naturally have a higher metabolism, making it easier to maintain or lose weight than others with a slower metabolism.

5. Muscle Mass: Muscle tissue requires more energy to maintain than fat tissue. Therefore, individuals with a higher proportion of lean muscle mass often have a higher metabolism. Strength training and resistance exercises can help increase muscle mass and boost metabolism.

6. Hormonal Influence: Hormones, such as thyroid hormones and insulin, play a role in regulating metabolism. Imbalances in these hormones can impact metabolic rate and, in turn, affect weight management.

The Roles Of Hormones In Metabolism

Hormones play critical roles in regulating various aspects of metabolism, influencing how the body uses and stores energy, and maintaining overall homeostasis. Different hormones act on other tissues and organs to coordinate metabolic processes. Understanding the interplay of these hormones is crucial for comprehending how the body regulates metabolism and energy balance. Hormonal imbalances can contribute to metabolic disorders, obesity, and other health issues, highlighting the importance of maintaining hormone balance for overall well-being.

Here are some key hormones and their roles in metabolism:

1. Insulin:

• Role: Insulin is produced by the pancreas and is essential for regulating blood glucose levels. It facilitates glucose uptake into cells, especially muscle and adipose (fat) cells, for energy use or storage.

• Effect on Metabolism: Insulin promotes the storage of excess glucose as glycogen in the liver and muscles. It also facilitates the conversion of glucose into fat in adipose tissue. Insulin helps lower blood sugar levels and promotes anabolic (building) processes.

1. Glucagon:

• Role: Also produced by the pancreas, glucagon has the opposite effect of insulin. It signals the release of glucose from the liver into the bloodstream when blood sugar levels are low.

• Effect on Metabolism: Glucagon stimulates glycogen breakdown in the liver, converting it into glucose. It also promotes the release of fatty acids from adipose tissue, making them available for energy production. Glucagon thus has a catabolic (breaking down) effect.

1. Cortisol:

• Role: The adrenal glands produce cortisol in response to stress, which is often called the "stress hormone." It plays a role in various functions, including regulating metabolism.

• Effect on Metabolism: Cortisol promotes the breakdown of proteins into amino acids and stimulates the conversion of amino acids into glucose (gluconeogenesis). It also enhances the release of fatty acids into the bloodstream, making more energy sources available during stressful situations.

1. Thyroid Hormones (T3 and T4):

• Role: Produced by the thyroid gland, thyroid hormones (triiodothyronine, T3, thyroxine, T4) are crucial for overall metabolism and energy regulation.

• Effect on Metabolism: Thyroid hormones increase the metabolic rate of cells, influencing the consumption of oxygen and the production of heat. They enhance the breakdown of nutrients for energy and help regulate body temperature.

1. Leptin:

• Role: Produced by adipose tissue, leptin acts as a satiety hormone, signaling to the brain that the body has sufficient energy stores.

• Effect on Metabolism: Leptin helps regulate energy balance by inhibiting hunger and promoting energy expenditure. In cases of obesity, leptin resistance can occur, leading to difficulties in appetite control.

1. Ghrelin:

• Role: Ghrelin is produced in the stomach and stimulates appetite.

• Effect on Metabolism: Ghrelin levels increase before meals, signaling hunger to the brain. It promotes food intake and reduces energy expenditure, playing a role in regulating body weight.

Common Metabolic Myths And Misconceptions

Several metabolic myths and misconceptions circulate in popular culture, often fueled by misinformation or misunderstandings about metabolism. Addressing these myths is essential for promoting accurate health information. Here are some common metabolic myths and the corresponding corrections:

Myth 1: Eating Late at Night Slows Down Your Metabolism

• Correction: The timing of meals doesn't significantly affect metabolism. The total amount of calories consumed versus expended throughout the day is more important for weight management. What matters most is the overall balance between caloric intake and expenditure.

Myth 2: Certain Foods Have Negative Calories

• Correction: There is no scientific basis for "negative-calorie" foods. While some foods may have a low-calorie content and require more energy to digest, the overall impact on metabolism is minimal. A balanced diet is crucial for health; no single food can magically lead to weight loss.

Myth 3: Drinking Ice-Cold Water Burns More Calories

• Correction: While it's true that the body expends some energy to warm cold water to body temperature, the calorie burn is minimal. Relying on this as a weight loss strategy could be more effective. Staying hydrated is essential, but the impact on metabolism is not significant in weight management.

Myth 4: Eating Spicy Foods Boosts Metabolism

• Correction: Some studies suggest that spicy foods, particularly those containing capsaicin, may have a modest, short-term effect on metabolism. However, this effect must be more substantial to lead to significant weight loss. A well-rounded diet and regular physical activity are more impactful for metabolic health.

Myth 5: Metabolism Slows Down Significantly with Age

• Correction: While there is a natural decline in metabolic rate with age, the decrease is often overestimated. Lifestyle factors, such as physical activity and muscle mass maintenance, play a more significant role in maintaining a healthy metabolism as individuals age.

Myth 6: Eating Small, Frequent Meals Boosts Metabolism

• Correction: The idea that eating multiple small meals throughout the day boosts metabolism is not universally supported by scientific evidence. Meal frequency can vary among individuals, and daily caloric intake remains crucial in weight management.

Myth 7: Detox Diets Boost Metabolism by Eliminating Toxins

• Correction: Scientific evidence does not support the concept of "detoxing" through restrictive diets or cleanses.

The body has its mechanisms for detoxification, primarily the liver and kidneys. Extreme diets can be harmful and do not provide long-term benefits for metabolic health.

12

◆ ◆ ◆

CHAPTER 2:

The Science Behind
Metabolic Confusion

The Concept Of Metabolic Adaptation

Metabolic adaptation is a fundamental principle that underlies the concept of Metabolic Confusion. Understanding how the body adjusts its energy expenditure in response to changes in caloric intake and physical activity is vital to appreciating the effectiveness of this innovative weight management approach.

In essence, metabolic adaptation within Metabolic Confusion is rooted in the idea that a dynamic and variable approach to diet and exercise prevents the body from settling into a state of metabolic complacency. By strategically implementing changes in caloric intake, macronutrient ratios, meal timing, and exercise patterns, individuals can promote a more adaptable metabolism, overcoming the challenges of conventional diets and fostering sustainable, long-term weight management.

1. Metabolic Set Point:

• Explanation: The body naturally maintains a stable weight, known as the metabolic set point. Various factors influence this set point, including genetics, hormonal regulation, and past weight history.

• Metabolic Adaptation: When individuals embark on a conventional diet with a consistent caloric deficit, the body may perceive this as a threat to its energy reserves. In response, metabolic adaptations occur to conserve energy, including a reduction in basal metabolic rate (BMR) and increased efficiency in nutrient utilization.

2. Caloric Cycling in Metabolic Confusion:

• Explanation: Metabolic Confusion introduces the concept of caloric cycling, where individuals alternate between higher and lower caloric intake periods. This cycling prevents the body from fully adapting to a prolonged caloric deficit, mitigating the harmful effects of metabolic slowdown.

• Metabolic Adaptation: By periodically providing the body with a higher caloric intake, Metabolic Confusion helps reset the metabolic set point. This prevents the body from downregulating its energy expenditure in response to a consistent caloric deficit, fostering a more flexible and adaptive metabolism.

3. Variability in Macronutrient Ratios:

• Explanation: In addition to caloric cycling, Metabolic Confusion involves varying macronutrient ratios. This approach challenges the body's metabolic flexibility, preventing it from becoming overly efficient in utilizing specific types of nutrients.

• Metabolic Adaptation: The variability in macronutrient ratios ensures that the body remains adaptable to different energy sources. This prevents metabolic staleness and enhances the metabolic rate by promoting the efficient utilization of carbohydrates and fats for energy.

4. Meal Timing and Frequency:

• Explanation: Metabolic Confusion also considers the timing and frequency of meals. Intermittent fasting or adjusting meal timing can influence hormones related to hunger and satiety, impacting overall energy balance.

• Metabolic Adaptation: By incorporating variations in meal timing and frequency, Metabolic Confusion disrupts predictable patterns, preventing the body from settling into a rigid metabolic routine. This can help regulate hormones like insulin and leptin, improving metabolic control.

5. Exercise as a Metabolic Stimulus:

• Explanation: Physical activity is a crucial component of Metabolic Confusion. Regular exercise, including cardiovascular and resistance training, is a metabolic stimulus contributing to overall metabolic flexibility.

• Metabolic Adaptation: Exercise induces metabolic adaptations by promoting the maintenance of lean muscle mass, increasing calorie expenditure, and influencing hormonal balance. This, in turn, supports a more responsive and efficient metabolism.

How changing your diet affects your metabolism

Changing your diet can have a significant impact on your metabolism. The metabolism is a dynamic and responsive system that adjusts based on the availability of nutrients and energy needs. Here's how changing your diet can affect your metabolism:

1. Caloric Intake:

• Effect: When you change your diet by altering the calories you consume, your body adjusts energy expenditure to maintain balance. If you reduce your caloric intake, your metabolism may slow down to conserve energy. Conversely, increasing caloric intake may lead to a temporary boost in metabolism.

• Consideration: Sustainable weight management often involves finding a balance between caloric intake and expenditure. Extreme caloric restriction can trigger metabolic adaptations, making long-term weight loss more challenging.

1. Macronutrient Composition:

• Effect: The types of macronutrients (carbohydrates, proteins, fats) in your diet influence metabolic processes differently. For example, protein requires more energy for digestion and can have a slight thermogenic effect, temporarily increasing calorie expenditure.

• Consideration: Balancing macronutrients is essential for overall health. Diets that excessively restrict one macronutrient may negatively impact metabolism and nutrient absorption.

1. Meal Timing and Frequency:

• Effect: The timing and frequency of meals can influence metabolism. Regular, spaced-out meals help maintain stable blood sugar levels and provide a steady energy supply, potentially preventing excessive fluctuations in metabolism.

• Consideration: Individual preferences and lifestyle factors play a role in determining the most suitable meal timing and frequency. Some people may benefit from intermittent fasting, while others may thrive with regular, evenly-spaced meals.

1. Nutrient Quality:

• Effect: The quality of nutrients in your diet influences metabolic health. Whole, nutrient-dense foods provide a broader range of essential vitamins and minerals that support metabolic functions.

• Consideration: Prioritize a diverse and balanced diet that includes a variety of fruits, vegetables, lean proteins, whole grains, and healthy fats to support overall metabolic well-being.

1. Hydration:

• Effect: Dehydration can temporarily reduce metabolic efficiency. Water is involved in various metabolic processes, and adequate hydration supports these functions.

• Consideration: Staying well-hydrated is crucial for overall health and can contribute to optimal metabolic function. Aim to drink enough water throughout the day.

1. Adaptations to Dietary Changes:

• Effect: The body adapts to dietary changes over time. For example, if you consistently consume a lower-carbohydrate diet, your body may become more efficient at using fats for energy.

• Consideration: Adaptations can be both positive and negative. While some adaptations may support weight loss or metabolic flexibility, extreme or unbalanced diets can lead to undesirable metabolic changes.

◆ ◆ ◆

CHAPTER 3:

The Principles of the
Metabolic Confusion Diet

The Metabolic Confusion Diet is based on principles that aim to promote a flexible and adaptive metabolism, prevent the body from plateauing, and optimise its ability to burn calories efficiently. Here are the key principles of the Metabolic Confusion Diet:

1. Caloric Cycling:

o Principle: The diet involves intentional variations in daily caloric intake, cycling between periods of higher and lower calorie consumption.

o Rationale: Caloric cycling prevents the body from adapting to a consistent calorie deficit, which can lead to metabolic slowdown. Alternating between higher and lower-calorie days helps maintain a more dynamic metabolism.

2. Variability in Macronutrient Ratios:

o Principle: The diet includes variations in the proportions of macronutrients (carbohydrates, proteins, and fats) consumed, rather than adhering to a fixed ratio.

o Rationale: Altering macronutrient ratios challenges the body's metabolic flexibility, preventing it from becoming overly efficient in utilising specific types of nutrients. This approach supports a more adaptable metabolism.

3. Intermittent Fasting or Meal Timing Variability:

o Principle: Incorporating intermittent fasting or varying meal timing introduces periods of fasting or eating within specific time windows.

o Rationale: Changes in meal timing and intermittent fasting can influence hormonal responses, such as insulin sensitivity and ghrelin levels. This variability may contribute to improved metabolic control.

4. Strategic Nutrient Manipulation:

o Principle: The diet involves strategically manipulating nutrient intake, such as carbohydrate cycling or adjusting nutrient timing in relation to physical activity.

o Rationale: By strategically manipulating nutrients, the diet aims to optimise energy availability for different metabolic processes. This can enhance performance during physical activity and support metabolic flexibility.

5. Incorporation of Regular Physical Activity:

o Principle: The Metabolic Confusion Diet emphasises the importance of regular exercise, including both cardiovascular and resistance training.

o Rationale: Exercise serves as a metabolic stimulus, promoting the maintenance of lean muscle mass, increasing calorie expenditure, and influencing hormonal balance. This supports an overall responsive and efficient metabolism.

6. Periodic Maintenance and Evaluation:

o Principle: The diet encourages periodic assessments and adjustments based on individual progress and goals.

o Rationale: Metabolic needs can change over time. Regular evaluations allow for adjustments to the diet plan, ensuring that it remains aligned with individual goals and promotes ongoing success.

7. Mindful Eating and Individualization:

o Principle: The Metabolic Confusion Diet encourages mindful eating and recognises the importance of individualization in dietary approaches.

o Rationale: Being attuned to hunger and satiety cues, as well as adapting the diet to individual preferences and lifestyles, enhances adherence and long-term sustainability.

8. Adequate Hydration:

o Principle: Staying well-hydrated is emphasised as a fundamental aspect of the diet.

o Rationale: Adequate hydration supports overall metabolic functions and can contribute to optimal physical and mental well-being.

Designing A Personalised Metabolic Confusion Plan

Designing a personalised metabolic confusion diet plan involves tailoring the principles of metabolic confusion to an individual's specific needs, preferences, and goals. Here's a step-by-step guide to help you create a personalised plan:

1. Assess the current status:

o Dietary Habits: Evaluate the individual's current eating patterns, including typical meals, snacks, and overall caloric intake.

o Physical Activity: Assess the individual's current exercise routine, including the type, frequency, and intensity of activities.

2. Set clear goals:

o Weight Management: Define specific, realistic, and measurable weight management goals, whether it's losing, maintaining, or gaining weight.

o Health Objectives: Consider other health goals, such as improving energy levels, managing blood sugar, or supporting muscle development.

3. Determine caloric needs:

o Calculate Basal Metabolic Rate (BMR): Use a reliable BMR calculator to estimate the number of calories the body needs at rest.

o Factor in Physical Activity: Adjust the BMR based on the individual's activity level to determine total daily energy expenditure (TDEE).

4. Implement calorie cycling:

o Higher Calorie Days: Designate days with a slight caloric surplus, emphasising nutrient-dense foods. This could coincide with more intense workout days.

o Lower-Calorie Days: Implement days with a caloric deficit, focusing on nutrient-dense, lower-calorie options. These days may align with rest or lighter activity days.

5. Adjust Macronutrient Ratios:

o Carbohydrates, proteins, and fats: Vary the proportions of macronutrients on different days. For example, emphasise carbohydrates on higher activity days and include more healthy fats on lower activity days.

o Consider Nutrient Timing: Adjust nutrient distribution throughout the day, considering pre- and post-workout nutrition.

6. Incorporate intermittent fasting or meal timing variability.

o Choose a method: Select an intermittent fasting approach or vary meal timing to introduce periods of fasting or eating within specific windows.

o Align with Lifestyle: Ensure the chosen method aligns with the individual's daily routine and preferences.

7. Strategic Nutrient Manipulation:

o Carbohydrate Cycling: If suitable, implement carbohydrate cycling by adjusting carbohydrate intake based on activity levels.

o Protein Timing: Consider spreading protein intake across meals, with a focus on post-workout protein to support muscle recovery.

8. Regular physical activity:

o Cardiovascular Exercise: Include regular cardiovascular activities, adjusting intensity based on the individual's fitness level.

o Resistance Training: Integrate resistance training to support muscle development and metabolic rate.

9. Periodic Maintenance and Adjustments:

o Regular Assessments: Schedule regular check-ins to evaluate progress, adjust caloric intake, and modify the diet plan as needed.

o Adapt to Changes: Be flexible and adapt the plan to accommodate changes in goals, preferences, or lifestyle.

10. Mindful Eating and Hydration:

o Mindful Practices: Encourage mindful eating, paying attention to hunger and fullness cues.

o Hydration: Emphasise the importance of staying well-hydrated throughout the day.

11. Consider individual preferences:

o Food Preferences: Design the plan around foods the individual enjoys to enhance adherence.

o Cultural Considerations: Respect cultural or personal dietary preferences when creating the plan.

Sample Meal Plans And Recipes

Creating sample meal plans and recipes for a Metabolic Confusion Diet involves incorporating variability in caloric intake, macronutrient ratios, and nutrient-dense foods.

Here are examples for a higher-calorie day, a lower-calorie day, and a workout day:

Higher Calorie Day:

Breakfast:

• Scrambled eggs with spinach and feta

• Whole-grain toast with avocado

• Greek yoghurt with berries

Lunch:

• Grilled chicken quinoa salad with a variety of colourful vegetables (bell peppers, cherry tomatoes, cucumber)

• Olive oil and balsamic vinegar dressing

Snack:

• A handful of almonds and walnuts

• Apple slices with peanut butter

Dinner:

• Baked salmon with sweet potato wedges

• Steamed broccoli and asparagus

• Quinoa or brown rice

Dessert:

• Dark chocolate and mixed berries

Lower Calorie Day:

Breakfast:

• Protein smoothie with almond milk, protein powder, and mixed berries

- Chia seed pudding

Lunch:

- Grilled chicken or tofu salad with mixed greens

- Cherry tomatoes, cucumber, and a light vinaigrette dressing

Snack:

- Carrot and celery sticks with hummus

Dinner:

- Stir-fried shrimp or tempeh with assorted vegetables (bell peppers, zucchini, mushrooms)

- Cauliflower rice or broccoli rice

Dessert:

- Fresh fruit salad

Workout Day:

Pre-Workout Snack:

- Banana with a tablespoon of almond butter

Post-Workout Meal:

- Protein-packed omelette with tomatoes, spinach, and cheese

- Whole-grain toast

Lunch:

- Quinoa bowl with grilled chicken or chickpeas, mixed vegetables, and a tahini dressing

Afternoon Snack:

- Cottage cheese with pineapple chunks

Dinner:

• Baked cod or tilapia with roasted sweet potatoes

• Steamed green beans

Evening Snack:

• Greek yoghurt with a drizzle of honey

Additional Tips:

• Hydration: Drink plenty of water throughout the day, and consider incorporating herbal teas or infused water for variety.

• Flexibility: Adapt portion sizes and ingredients based on individual preferences and dietary needs.

• Experimentation: Encourage trying new recipes and exploring a variety of foods to keep the diet interesting.

$$\blacklozenge \; \blacklozenge \; \blacklozenge$$

CHAPTER 4:

Metabolic Confusion Diet Recipes

Welcome to the kitchen of metabolic adaptation, where we embrace the diverse flavors and nourishing ingredients that fuel the journey toward a balanced and responsive metabolism. The Metabolic Confusion Diet is not just a list of rules; it's a culinary adventure that celebrates variability, mindfulness, and the pleasure of eating for optimal well-being.

Breakfasts to Ignite Your Day:

Metabolic Boost Smoothie

Ingredients:

• 1 cup spinach leaves, washed

• 1 cup kale leaves, stems removed

• 1 ripe banana, peeled

• 1/2 cup Greek yogurt

• 1 cup unsweetened almond milk

• 1 tablespoon chia seeds

Instructions:

1. Prepare Ingredients:

o Wash the spinach and kale thoroughly.

o Peel the ripe banana.

2. Assemble in Blender:

o In a blender, add the spinach, kale, banana, Greek yogurt, almond milk, and chia seeds.

3. Blend Until Smooth:

o Blend the ingredients on high speed until you achieve a smooth and creamy consistency.

4. Adjust Consistency (Optional):

o If the smoothie is too thick, you can add more almond milk in small increments until you reach your desired consistency.

5. Serve and Enjoy:

o Pour the smoothie into a glass or a portable cup.

6. Garnish (Optional):

o Garnish with a sprinkle of additional chia seeds or a slice of banana if desired.

7. Nutritional Information (Per Serving):

o Calories: Approximately 250 kcal

o Protein: 15g

o Fat: 8g

o Carbohydrates: 35g

o Fiber: 9g

o Sugar: 15g

Note:

• This Metabolic Boost Smoothie is a nutrient-packed powerhouse, rich in vitamins, minerals, and antioxidants.

• The combination of spinach and kale provides a generous dose of iron, vitamin K, vitamin A, and folate.

• Greek yogurt contributes protein and probiotics for gut health.

• Almond milk adds creaminess without dairy, suitable for those with lactose intolerance.

• Chia seeds provide omega-3 fatty acids, fiber, and a satisfying texture.

• This smoothie can serve as a quick and nutritious breakfast or a refreshing snack, contributing to a dynamic and adaptable metabolism.

Protein-Packed Omelet with Avocado

Ingredients:

• 3 large eggs

• 1/4 cup diced bell peppers (mix of colors)

• 2 tablespoons diced onions

- 1/4 cup cherry tomatoes, halved
- 2 tablespoons crumbled feta cheese
- 1/2 ripe avocado, sliced
- Salt and pepper to taste
- 1 tablespoon olive oil (for cooking)

Instructions:

1. Prepare Vegetables:

o Dice the bell peppers and onions.

o Halve the cherry tomatoes.

o Crumble the feta cheese.

2. Whisk Eggs:

o In a bowl, crack the eggs and whisk them until well combined.

o Season with a pinch of salt and pepper.

3. Preheat Pan:

o Heat olive oil in a non-stick skillet over medium heat.

4. Sauté Vegetables:

o Add diced bell peppers and onions to the pan.

o Sauté until the vegetables are softened, about 2-3 minutes.

5. Add Eggs to the Pan:

o Pour the whisked eggs over the sautéed vegetables in the pan.

6. Cook the Omelet:

o Allow the eggs to set slightly at the edges.

o Gently lift the edges of the omelet with a spatula,

allowing uncooked eggs to flow underneath.

7. Add Tomatoes and Feta:

o Sprinkle halved cherry tomatoes and crumbled feta cheese over one half of the omelet.

8. Fold and Serve:

o Once the eggs are mostly set but still slightly runny on top, fold the omelet in half using the spatula.

o Continue cooking for an additional 1-2 minutes until the cheese melts, and the omelet is cooked through.

9. Plate and Garnish:

o Carefully transfer the omelet to a plate.

o Top with sliced avocado.

10. Season and Serve:

o Season the omelet with additional salt and pepper if needed.

o Serve immediately, and enjoy your protein-packed omelet with creamy avocado.

Nutritional Information (Per Serving):

• Calories: Approximately 350 kcal

• Protein: 20g

• Fat: 25g

• Carbohydrates: 12g

• Fiber: 5g

• Sugar: 3g

Note:

• This Protein-Packed Omelet with Avocado is a balanced

and satiating meal, providing a good source of protein, healthy fats, and essential nutrients.

• Bell peppers and tomatoes contribute vitamins C and A, while onions add flavor and additional nutrients.

• Feta cheese offers a tangy kick and a dose of calcium.

• Avocado adds creaminess and heart-healthy monounsaturated fats.

• This omelet is suitable for breakfast, brunch, or a quick and nutritious dinner, supporting your metabolic health with a delicious and satisfying combination of ingredients.

Quinoa Power Bowl

Ingredients:

• 1 cup quinoa, rinsed

• 1 cup grilled chicken breast, shredded (or 1 cup cooked chickpeas for a vegetarian option)

• 1 cup broccoli florets

• 1/2 cup carrots, julienned

• 1/2 cup bell peppers (mix of colors), sliced

• 2 tablespoons tahini dressing (see below for ingredients)

• Salt and pepper to taste

• Olive oil for cooking

Tahini Dressing:

• 3 tablespoons tahini

• 2 tablespoons lemon juice

- 2 tablespoons water

- 1 clove garlic, minced

- Salt and pepper to taste

Instructions:

Quinoa:

1. Rinse Quinoa:

o Rinse quinoa under cold water to remove any bitterness.

2. Cook Quinoa:

o In a medium saucepan, combine 1 cup of rinsed quinoa with 2 cups of water.

o Bring to a boil, then reduce heat to low, cover, and simmer for 15-20 minutes or until the quinoa is cooked and water is absorbed.

o Fluff with a fork.

Grilled Chicken:

3. Season and Grill Chicken:

o Season chicken breasts with salt and pepper.

o Grill until fully cooked, about 4-6 minutes per side.

o Shred the grilled chicken using two forks.

Tahini Dressing:

4. Prepare Tahini Dressing:

o In a small bowl, whisk together tahini, lemon juice, water, minced garlic, salt, and pepper until well combined.

o Adjust the consistency with more water if needed.

Vegetables:

5. Sauté Vegetables:

o In a separate pan, heat olive oil over medium heat.

o Sauté broccoli, carrots, and bell peppers until tender-crisp, about 5-7 minutes.

o Season with salt and pepper.

Assembling the Quinoa Power Bowl:

6. Arrange Components:

o In serving bowls, arrange a portion of cooked quinoa, grilled chicken or chickpeas, and sautéed vegetables.

7. Drizzle with Tahini Dressing:

o Drizzle the tahini dressing over the quinoa, chicken, and vegetables.

8. Toss and Serve:

o Gently toss the components together to coat them in the dressing.

9. Nutritional Information (Per Serving):

o Calories: Approximately 450 kcal

o Protein: 25g

o Fat: 18g

o Carbohydrates: 50g

o Fiber: 8g

o Sugar: 3g

Note:

• This Quinoa Power Bowl is a nutrient-dense and balanced

meal, offering a combination of whole grains, lean protein, and colorful vegetables.

• Quinoa provides a complete protein source, and the tahini dressing adds healthy fats and a flavorful kick.

• Customize the bowl with your favorite vegetables or add a squeeze of lemon for extra freshness.

• Enjoy this versatile and satisfying bowl for lunch or dinner, supporting your metabolic health with a variety of wholesome ingredients.

Mediterranean Salad Delight

Ingredients:

• 4 cups mixed greens (e.g., spinach, arugula, romaine)

• 1 cup cherry tomatoes, halved

• 1 cucumber, sliced

• 1/2 cup Kalamata olives, pitted

• 1/2 cup crumbled feta cheese

• 8 ounces grilled shrimp (or grilled tofu for a vegetarian option)

• Olive oil for drizzling

• Balsamic vinegar for dressing

• Salt and pepper to taste

• Fresh lemon wedges for serving

Instructions:

Grilled Shrimp or Tofu:

1. Prepare Protein:

o If using shrimp, season them with salt, pepper, and a drizzle of olive oil. Grill until opaque and cooked through (about 2-3 minutes per side).

o If using tofu, press and cut it into cubes. Grill or sauté until golden brown on all sides.

Assembling the Salad:

2. Prepare Vegetables: o Wash and chop the mixed greens, halve the cherry tomatoes, slice the cucumber, and pit the olives if necessary.

3. Assemble the Base:

o In a large salad bowl, arrange the mixed greens as the base.

4. Layer Vegetables:

o Scatter cherry tomatoes, cucumber slices, Kalamata olives, and crumbled feta cheese over the greens.

5. Add Grilled Protein:

o Place the grilled shrimp or tofu on top of the salad.

6. Drizzle with Dressing:

o Drizzle olive oil and balsamic vinegar over the salad.

7. Toss Gently:

o Toss the salad gently to evenly distribute the ingredients.

8. Season to Taste:

o Season with salt and pepper to taste.

9. Serve and Garnish:

o Serve the salad in individual bowls or on a platter.

o Garnish with additional feta cheese if desired.

10. Nutritional Information (Per Serving):

o Calories: Approximately 300 kcal

o Protein: 20g

o Fat: 15g

o Carbohydrates: 20g

o Fiber: 5g

o Sugar: 8g

Note:

• This Mediterranean Salad Delight is a refreshing and nutrient-dense meal inspired by the flavors of the Mediterranean diet.

• The combination of mixed greens, colorful vegetables, olives, and feta cheese provides a variety of vitamins, minerals, and antioxidants.

• Grilled shrimp or tofu adds a protein boost, making this salad a satisfying and balanced dish.

• Drizzle with olive oil and balsamic vinegar for a simple and flavorful dressing.

• Enjoy this salad as a light lunch or dinner, promoting metabolic well-being through a diverse array of wholesome ingredients.

Nutty Apple Slices

Ingredients:

• 2 medium-sized apples, cored and sliced

• 1/4 cup almond butter

• 1/4 cup walnuts, crushed

Instructions:

1. Prepare Apples:

o Wash, core, and slice the apples into thin rounds.

2. Crush Walnuts:

o Place the walnuts in a sealed plastic bag and crush them using a rolling pin or the back of a heavy utensil.

3. Assemble Apple Slices:

o Lay the apple slices on a serving plate or individual plates.

4. Spread Almond Butter:

o Using a butter knife or spoon, spread a thin layer of almond butter onto each apple slice.

5. Sprinkle Crushed Walnuts:

o Sprinkle the crushed walnuts over the almond butter-covered apple slices.

6. Serve and Enjoy:

o Arrange the Nutty Apple Slices on a serving platter or individual plates.

7. Nutritional Information (Per Serving):

o Calories: Approximately 200 kcal

o Protein: 4g

o Fat: 12g

o Carbohydrates: 22g

o Fiber: 5g

o Sugar: 15g

Note:

• Nutty Apple Slices make for a delicious and nutritious snack that balances natural sweetness with healthy fats and protein.

• Apples provide dietary fiber, while almond butter adds protein and healthy fats.

• Walnuts contribute omega-3 fatty acids and a satisfying crunch.

• This snack is quick to prepare and is an excellent option for a midday energy boost or a sweet and wholesome dessert.

• Adjust the quantities based on your preferences and dietary needs, and enjoy the delightful combination of flavors and textures.

Stir-Fried Tofu with Rainbow Vegetables

Ingredients:

• 14 oz (400g) firm tofu, pressed and cubed

• 1 red bell pepper, thinly sliced

• 1 yellow bell pepper, thinly sliced

• 1 zucchini, thinly sliced

• 1 cup broccoli florets

• 2 tablespoons soy sauce

• 2 tablespoons vegetable oil

- 1 teaspoon sesame oil (optional)
- 1 tablespoon fresh ginger, minced
- 2 cloves garlic, minced
- Green onions for garnish (optional)
- Sesame seeds for garnish (optional)

Instructions:

1. Press Tofu:

o Place the block of tofu on a plate with paper towels underneath and on top. Press with a heavy object for at least 30 minutes to remove excess moisture.

2. Cube Tofu:

o Cut the pressed tofu into 1-inch cubes.

3. Prepare Vegetables:

o Slice the bell peppers, zucchini, and thinly chop the broccoli florets.

4. Heat Pan:

o Heat vegetable oil in a large pan or wok over medium-high heat.

5. Sauté Tofu:

o Add the cubed tofu to the hot pan and stir-fry until golden brown on all sides, about 5-7 minutes.

6. Add Vegetables:

o Add the sliced bell peppers, zucchini, and broccoli to the pan. Stir-fry for an additional 5-7 minutes until the vegetables are tender-crisp.

7. Prepare Sauce:

o In a small bowl, mix soy sauce, sesame oil (if using),

minced ginger, and minced garlic.

8. Combine Sauce:

o Pour the sauce over the tofu and vegetables. Toss everything together to ensure an even coating.

9. Finish Cooking:

o Continue to stir-fry for an additional 2-3 minutes, allowing the flavors to meld and the sauce to thicken slightly.

10. Garnish and Serve:

o Garnish with chopped green onions and sesame seeds if desired.

11. Nutritional Information (Per Serving):

o Calories: Approximately 300 kcal

o Protein: 18g

o Fat: 20g

o Carbohydrates: 15g

o Fiber: 5g

o Sugar: 5g

Note:

• Stir-Fried Tofu with Rainbow Vegetables is a colorful and nutrient-packed dish that combines the protein of tofu with the vitamins and minerals of various vegetables.

• Pressing the tofu ensures a firmer texture and better absorption of flavors.

• Feel free to customize the vegetables based on personal

preferences or seasonal availability.

• Serve over brown rice or quinoa for a complete and satisfying meal that supports metabolic health through a diverse array of plant-based nutrients.

•

Energizing Lunch Creations:

Quinoa Power Bowl

Ingredients:

For the Quinoa:

• 1 cup quinoa, rinsed

• 2 cups water

• Pinch of salt

For the Grilled Chicken:

• 1 pound (about 450g) boneless, skinless chicken breasts

• 1 tablespoon olive oil

• Salt and pepper to taste

• 1 teaspoon paprika

• 1 teaspoon garlic powder

For the Chickpeas (Vegetarian Option):

• 1 can (15 oz) chickpeas, drained and rinsed

• 1 tablespoon olive oil

• 1 teaspoon cumin

• 1 teaspoon smoked paprika

• Salt and pepper to taste

For the Mixed Vegetables:

• 2 cups broccoli florets

• 1 cup carrots, julienned

• 1 cup bell peppers (mix of colors), sliced

• 2 tablespoons olive oil

• Salt and pepper to taste

For the Tahini Dressing:

• 1/4 cup tahini

• 2 tablespoons lemon juice

• 2 tablespoons water

• 1 clove garlic, minced

• Salt and pepper to taste

Instructions:

Quinoa:

1. Rinse Quinoa:

o Rinse quinoa under cold water to remove any bitterness.

2. Cook Quinoa:

o In a medium saucepan, combine 1 cup rinsed quinoa, 2 cups water, and a pinch of salt.

o Bring to a boil, then reduce heat to low, cover, and simmer for 15-20 minutes or until the quinoa is cooked and water is absorbed.

o Fluff with a fork.

Grilled Chicken:

3. Prepare Chicken:

o Season chicken breasts with salt, pepper, paprika, and garlic powder.

o In a skillet, heat olive oil over medium-high heat.

o Grill the chicken for 6-8 minutes per side or until fully cooked.

Chickpeas (Vegetarian Option):

4. Prepare Chickpeas:

o In a skillet, heat olive oil over medium heat.

o Add chickpeas, cumin, smoked paprika, salt, and pepper.

o Sauté for 5-7 minutes until chickpeas are golden and coated with spices.

Mixed Vegetables:

5. Sauté Vegetables:

o In a separate pan, heat olive oil over medium heat.

o Add broccoli, carrots, and bell peppers.

o Sauté for 7-10 minutes until vegetables are tender-crisp.

o Season with salt and pepper.

Tahini Dressing:

6. Prepare Tahini Dressing:

o In a small bowl, whisk together tahini, lemon juice, water, minced garlic, salt, and pepper.

o Adjust the consistency with more water if needed.

Assembling the Quinoa Power Bowl:

7. Assemble Components:

o In serving bowls, arrange a portion of cooked quinoa, grilled chicken or chickpeas, and sautéed mixed vegetables.

8. Drizzle with Tahini Dressing:

o Drizzle the tahini dressing over the quinoa, protein, and vegetables.

9. Nutritional Information (Per Serving):

o Calories: Approximately 500 kcal

o Protein: 25g

o Fat: 20g

o Carbohydrates: 50g

o Fiber: 10g

o Sugar: 5g

Note:

• The Quinoa Power Bowl is a well-rounded and nutrient-dense meal, combining whole grains, lean protein, and colorful vegetables.

• The tahini dressing adds a creamy and flavorful touch while contributing healthy fats.

• Customize the bowl with your favorite vegetables or protein sources.

• Enjoy this bowl for lunch or dinner, supporting metabolic health with a diverse array of wholesome ingredients.

Mediterranean Salad Delight

Ingredients:

For the Salad:

• 4 cups mixed greens (e.g., spinach, arugula, romaine)

• 1 cup cherry tomatoes, halved

• 1 cucumber, sliced

• 1/2 cup Kalamata olives, pitted

• 1/2 cup crumbled feta cheese

• 8 ounces grilled shrimp (or grilled tofu for a vegetarian option)

For the Dressing:

• 3 tablespoons extra virgin olive oil

• 2 tablespoons red wine vinegar

• 1 teaspoon Dijon mustard

• 1 clove garlic, minced

• Salt and pepper to taste

• 1 teaspoon dried oregano (optional)

Instructions:

Grilled Shrimp or Tofu:

1. Prepare Protein:

o If using shrimp, season them with salt, pepper, and a drizzle of olive oil. Grill until opaque and cooked through (about 2-3 minutes per side).

o If using tofu, press and cut it into cubes. Grill or sauté until golden brown on all sides.

Assembling the Salad:

2. Prepare Vegetables:

o Wash and chop the mixed greens, halve the cherry tomatoes, slice the cucumber, and pit the olives if necessary.

3. Assemble the Base:

o In a large salad bowl, arrange the mixed greens as the base.

4. Layer Vegetables:

o Scatter cherry tomatoes, cucumber slices, Kalamata olives, and crumbled feta cheese over the greens.

5. Add Grilled Protein:

o Place the grilled shrimp or tofu on top of the salad.

Dressing:

6. Prepare Dressing:

o In a small bowl, whisk together olive oil, red wine vinegar, Dijon mustard, minced garlic, salt, pepper, and dried oregano if using.

7. Drizzle Dressing:

o Drizzle the dressing over the salad. Toss gently to combine.

8. Serve and Enjoy:

o Serve the salad in individual bowls or on a platter.

9. Nutritional Information (Per Serving):

o Calories: Approximately 350 kcal

o Protein: 20g

o Fat: 18g

o Carbohydrates: 20g

o Fiber: 5g

o Sugar: 8g

Note:

• This Mediterranean Salad Delight is a vibrant and nutrient-packed dish inspired by the flavors of the Mediterranean diet.

• The combination of mixed greens, colorful vegetables, olives, and feta cheese provides a variety of vitamins, minerals, and antioxidants.

• Grilled shrimp or tofu adds a protein boost, making this salad a satisfying and balanced meal.

• The homemade dressing enhances the flavors with a perfect blend of acidity and savory notes.

• Enjoy this salad as a refreshing and wholesome lunch or dinner option, supporting your metabolic health with a diverse array of nutritious ingredients.

Metabolic Boost Smoothie

Ingredients:

• 1 cup spinach leaves, washed

• 1 cup kale leaves, stems removed

• 1 ripe banana, peeled

• 1/2 cup Greek yogurt

• 1 cup unsweetened almond milk

• 1 tablespoon chia seeds

Instructions:

1. Prepare Ingredients:

o Wash the spinach and kale thoroughly.

o Peel the ripe banana.

2. Assemble in Blender:

o In a blender, add the spinach, kale, banana, Greek yogurt, almond milk, and chia seeds.

3. Blend Until Smooth:

o Blend the ingredients on high speed until you achieve a smooth and creamy consistency.

4. Adjust Consistency (Optional):

o If the smoothie is too thick, you can add more almond milk in small increments until you reach your desired consistency.

5. Serve and Enjoy:

o Pour the smoothie into a glass or a portable cup.

6. Garnish (Optional):

o Garnish with a sprinkle of additional chia seeds or a slice of banana if desired.

7. Nutritional Information (Per Serving):

o Calories: Approximately 250 kcal

o Protein: 15g

o Fat: 8g

o Carbohydrates: 35g

o Fiber: 9g

o Sugar: 15g

Note:

• This Metabolic Boost Smoothie is a nutrient-packed

powerhouse, rich in vitamins, minerals, and antioxidants.

• The combination of spinach and kale provides a generous dose of iron, vitamin K, vitamin A, and folate.

• Greek yogurt contributes protein and probiotics for gut health.

• Almond milk adds creaminess without dairy, suitable for those with lactose intolerance.

• Chia seeds provide omega-3 fatty acids, fiber, and a satisfying texture.

• This smoothie can serve as a quick and nutritious breakfast or a refreshing snack, contributing to a dynamic and adaptable metabolism.

Protein-Packed Omelet with Avocado

Ingredients:

• 3 large eggs

• 1/4 cup diced bell peppers (mix of colors)

• 2 tablespoons diced onions

• 1/4 cup cherry tomatoes, halved

• 2 tablespoons crumbled feta cheese

• 1/2 ripe avocado, sliced

• Salt and pepper to taste

• 1 tablespoon olive oil (for cooking)

Instructions:

1. Prepare Vegetables:

o Dice the bell peppers and onions.

o Halve the cherry tomatoes.

o Crumble the feta cheese.

2. Whisk Eggs:

o In a bowl, crack the eggs and whisk them until well combined.

o Season with a pinch of salt and pepper.

3. Preheat Pan:

o Heat olive oil in a non-stick skillet over medium heat.

4. Sauté Vegetables:

o Add diced bell peppers and onions to the pan.

o Sauté until the vegetables are softened, about 2-3 minutes.

5. Add Eggs to the Pan:

o Pour the whisked eggs over the sautéed vegetables in the pan.

6. Cook the Omelet:

o Allow the eggs to set slightly at the edges.

o Gently lift the edges of the omelet with a spatula, allowing uncooked eggs to flow underneath.

7. Add Tomatoes and Feta:

o Sprinkle halved cherry tomatoes and crumbled feta cheese over one half of the omelet.

8. Fold and Serve:

o Once the eggs are mostly set but still slightly runny on top, fold the omelet in half using the spatula.

o Continue cooking for an additional 1-2 minutes until the cheese melts, and the omelet is cooked through.

9. Plate and Garnish:

o Carefully transfer the omelet to a plate.

o Top with sliced avocado.

10. Season and Serve:

o Season the omelet with additional salt and pepper if needed.

o Serve immediately, and enjoy your protein-packed omelet with creamy avocado.

Nutritional Information (Per Serving):

• Calories: Approximately 350 kcal

• Protein: 20g

• Fat: 25g

• Carbohydrates: 12g

• Fiber: 5g

• Sugar: 3g

Note:

• This Protein-Packed Omelet with Avocado is a balanced and satiating meal, providing a good source of protein, healthy fats, and essential nutrients.

• Bell peppers and tomatoes contribute vitamins C and A, while onions add flavor and additional nutrients.

• Feta cheese offers a tangy kick and a dose of calcium.

• Avocado adds creaminess and heart-healthy monounsaturated fats.

• This omelet is suitable for breakfast, brunch, or a quick

and nutritious dinner, supporting your metabolic health with a delicious and satisfying combination of ingredients.

Nutty Apple Slices

Ingredients:

• 2 medium-sized apples, cored and sliced

• 1/4 cup almond butter

• 1/4 cup walnuts, crushed

Instructions:

1. Prepare Apples:

o Wash, core, and slice the apples into thin rounds.

2. Crush Walnuts:

o Place the walnuts in a sealed plastic bag and crush them using a rolling pin or the back of a heavy utensil.

3. Assemble Apple Slices:

o Lay the apple slices on a serving plate or individual plates.

4. Spread Almond Butter:

o Using a butter knife or spoon, spread a thin layer of almond butter onto each apple slice.

5. Sprinkle Crushed Walnuts:

o Sprinkle the crushed walnuts over the almond butter-covered apple slices.

6. Serve and Enjoy:

o Arrange the Nutty Apple Slices on a serving platter or individual plates.

Nutritional Information (Per Serving):

• Calories: Approximately 200 kcal

• Protein: 4g

• Fat: 12g

• Carbohydrates: 22g

• Fiber: 5g

• Sugar: 15g

Note:

• Nutty Apple Slices make for a delicious and nutritious snack that balances natural sweetness with healthy fats and protein.

• Apples provide dietary fiber, while almond butter adds protein and healthy fats.

• Walnuts contribute omega-3 fatty acids and a satisfying crunch.

• This snack is quick to prepare and is an excellent option for a midday energy boost or a sweet and wholesome dessert.

• Adjust the quantities based on your preferences and dietary needs, and enjoy the delightful combination of flavors and textures.

Stir-Fried Tofu with Rainbow Vegetables

Ingredients:

For the Stir-Fry:

• 14 oz (400g) firm tofu, pressed and cubed

• 1 red bell pepper, thinly sliced

• 1 yellow bell pepper, thinly sliced

• 1 zucchini, thinly sliced

• 1 cup broccoli florets

• 2 tablespoons soy sauce

• 2 tablespoons vegetable oil

• 1 teaspoon sesame oil (optional)

• 1 tablespoon fresh ginger, minced

• 2 cloves garlic, minced

• Green onions for garnish (optional)

• Sesame seeds for garnish (optional)

Instructions:

1. Press Tofu:

o Place the block of tofu on a plate with paper towels underneath and on top. Press with a heavy object for at least 30 minutes to remove excess moisture.

2. Cube Tofu:

o Cut the pressed tofu into 1-inch cubes.

3. Prepare Vegetables:

o Slice the bell peppers, zucchini, and thinly chop the broccoli florets.

4. Heat Pan:

o Heat vegetable oil in a large pan or wok over medium-high heat.

5. Sauté Tofu:

o Add the cubed tofu to the hot pan and stir-fry until golden brown on all sides, about 5-7 minutes.

6. Add Vegetables:

o Add sliced bell peppers, zucchini, and broccoli to the pan. Stir-fry for an additional 5-7 minutes until the vegetables are tender-crisp.

7. Prepare Sauce:

o In a small bowl, mix soy sauce, sesame oil (if using), minced ginger, and minced garlic.

8. Combine Sauce:

o Pour the sauce over the tofu and vegetables. Toss everything together to ensure an even coating.

9. Finish Cooking:

o Continue to stir-fry for an additional 2-3 minutes,

allowing the flavors to meld and the sauce to thicken slightly.

10. Garnish and Serve:

o Garnish with chopped green onions and sesame seeds if desired.

Nutritional Information (Per Serving):

• Calories: Approximately 300 kcal

• Protein: 18g

• Fat: 20g

• Carbohydrates: 15g

• Fiber: 5g

• Sugar: 5g

Note:

• Stir-Fried Tofu with Rainbow Vegetables is a colorful and nutrient-packed dish that combines the protein of tofu with the vitamins and minerals of various vegetables.

• Pressing the tofu ensures a firmer texture and better absorption of flavors.

• Feel free to customize the vegetables based on personal preferences or seasonal availability.

• Serve over brown rice or quinoa for a complete and satisfying meal that supports metabolic health through a diverse array of plant-based nutrients.

•

Flavorful Snacks to Satisfy:

Nutty Apple Slices

Ingredients:

• 2 medium-sized apples, cored and sliced

• 1/4 cup almond butter

• 1/4 cup walnuts, crushed

Instructions:

1. Prepare Apples:

o Wash, core, and slice the apples into thin rounds.

2. Crush Walnuts:

o Place the walnuts in a sealed plastic bag and crush them using a rolling pin or the back of a heavy utensil.

3. Assemble Apple Slices:

o Lay the apple slices on a serving plate or individual plates.

4. Spread Almond Butter:

o Using a butter knife or spoon, spread a thin layer of almond butter onto each apple slice.

5. Sprinkle Crushed Walnuts:

o Sprinkle the crushed walnuts over the almond butter-covered apple slices.

6. Serve and Enjoy:

o Arrange the Nutty Apple Slices on a serving platter or individual plates.

Nutritional Information (Per Serving):

• Calories: Approximately 200 kcal

• Protein: 4g

• Fat: 12g

- Carbohydrates: 22g
- Fiber: 5g
- Sugar: 15g

Note:

- Nutty Apple Slices make for a delicious and nutritious snack that balances natural sweetness with healthy fats and protein.

- Apples provide dietary fiber, while almond butter adds protein and healthy fats.

- Walnuts contribute omega-3 fatty acids and a satisfying crunch.

- This snack is quick to prepare and is an excellent option for a midday energy boost or a sweet and wholesome dessert.

- Adjust the quantities based on your preferences and dietary needs, and enjoy the delightful combination of flavors and textures.

Veggies and Hummus Platter

Ingredients:

For the Platter:

- Carrot sticks
- Celery sticks
- Cherry tomatoes
- Cucumber, sliced

• Hummus

Instructions:

1. Prepare Vegetables:

o Wash and peel (if necessary) the carrots and cucumber.

o Cut the carrots and cucumbers into sticks.

o Cut celery into sticks.

2. Arrange on Platter:

o Arrange the carrot sticks, celery sticks, cherry tomatoes, and cucumber slices on a serving platter.

3. Place Hummus:

o Place a bowl or several smaller bowls of hummus in the center of the platter.

4. Garnish (Optional):

o Optionally, garnish the platter with fresh herbs or a drizzle of olive oil for added flavor and presentation.

5. Serve and Enjoy:

o Serve the Veggies and Hummus Platter at room temperature.

Nutritional Information (Per Serving):

• Calories: Approximately 150 kcal

• Protein: 5g

• Fat: 8g

• Carbohydrates: 18g

• Fiber: 6g

• Sugar: 5g

Note:

• The Veggies and Hummus Platter is a nutritious and satisfying snack or appetizer, perfect for sharing.

• Carrots provide beta-carotene, cucumber adds hydration, and celery contributes crunch.

• Cherry tomatoes are rich in antioxidants and add a burst of freshness.

• Hummus, made from chickpeas, provides protein and healthy fats, making this platter a well-balanced and metabolism-friendly option.

• Customize the platter with your favorite vegetables and hummus variations for a delicious and wholesome experience.

Metabolic Boost Smoothie

Ingredients:

• 1 cup spinach leaves, washed

• 1 cup kale leaves, stems removed

• 1 ripe banana, peeled

• 1/2 cup Greek yogurt

• 1 cup unsweetened almond milk

• 1 tablespoon chia seeds

Instructions:

1. Prepare Ingredients:

o Wash the spinach and kale thoroughly.

o Peel the ripe banana.

2. Assemble in Blender:

o In a blender, add the spinach, kale, banana, Greek yogurt, almond milk, and chia seeds.

3. Blend Until Smooth:

o Blend the ingredients on high speed until you achieve a smooth and creamy consistency.

4. Adjust Consistency (Optional):

o If the smoothie is too thick, you can add more almond milk in small increments until you reach your desired consistency.

5. Serve and Enjoy:

o Pour the smoothie into a glass or a portable cup.

6. Garnish (Optional):

o Garnish with a sprinkle of additional chia seeds or a slice of banana if desired.

7. Nutritional Information (Per Serving):

o Calories: Approximately 250 kcal

o Protein: 15g

o Fat: 8g

o Carbohydrates: 35g

o Fiber: 9g

o Sugar: 15g

Note:

• This Metabolic Boost Smoothie is a nutrient-packed powerhouse, rich in vitamins, minerals, and antioxidants.

• The combination of spinach and kale provides a generous dose of iron, vitamin K, vitamin A, and folate.

• Greek yogurt contributes protein and probiotics for gut

health.

• Almond milk adds creaminess without dairy, suitable for those with lactose intolerance.

• Chia seeds provide omega-3 fatty acids, fiber, and a satisfying texture.

• This smoothie can serve as a quick and nutritious breakfast or a refreshing snack, contributing to a dynamic and adaptable metabolism.

Protein-Packed Omelet with Avocado

Ingredients:

• 3 large eggs

• 1/4 cup diced bell peppers (mix of colors)

• 2 tablespoons diced onions

• 1/4 cup cherry tomatoes, halved

• 2 tablespoons crumbled feta cheese

• 1/2 ripe avocado, sliced

• Salt and pepper to taste

• 1 tablespoon olive oil (for cooking)

Instructions:

1. Prepare Vegetables:

o Dice the bell peppers and onions.

o Halve the cherry tomatoes.

o Crumble the feta cheese.

2. Whisk Eggs:

o In a bowl, crack the eggs and whisk them until well combined.

o Season with a pinch of salt and pepper.

3. Preheat Pan:

o Heat olive oil in a non-stick skillet over medium heat.

4. Sauté Vegetables:

o Add diced bell peppers and onions to the pan.

o Sauté until the vegetables are softened, about 2-3 minutes.

5. Add Eggs to the Pan:

o Pour the whisked eggs over the sautéed vegetables in the pan.

6. Cook the Omelet:

o Allow the eggs to set slightly at the edges.

o Gently lift the edges of the omelet with a spatula, allowing uncooked eggs to flow underneath.

7. Add Tomatoes and Feta:

o Sprinkle halved cherry tomatoes and crumbled feta cheese over one half of the omelet.

8. Fold and Serve:

o Once the eggs are mostly set but still slightly runny on top, fold the omelet in half using the spatula.

o Continue cooking for an additional 1-2 minutes until the cheese melts, and the omelet is cooked through.

9. Plate and Garnish:

o Carefully transfer the omelet to a plate.

o Top with sliced avocado.

10. Season and Serve:

o Season the omelet with additional salt and pepper if needed.

o Serve immediately, and enjoy your protein-packed omelet with creamy avocado.

Nutritional Information (Per Serving):

• Calories: Approximately 350 kcal

• Protein: 20g

• Fat: 25g

• Carbohydrates: 12g

• Fiber: 5g

• Sugar: 3g

Note:

• This Protein-Packed Omelet with Avocado is a balanced and satiating meal, providing a good source of protein, healthy fats, and essential nutrients.

• Bell peppers and tomatoes contribute vitamins C and A, while onions add flavor and additional nutrients.

• Feta cheese offers a tangy kick and a dose of calcium.

• Avocado adds creaminess and heart-healthy monounsaturated fats.

• This omelet is suitable for breakfast, brunch, or a quick and nutritious dinner, supporting your metabolic health with a delicious and satisfying combination of ingredients.

Quinoa Power Bowl

Ingredients:

For the Bowl:

• 1 cup quinoa, uncooked

• Grilled chicken breast strips or cooked chickpeas

• Mixed vegetables (broccoli florets, sliced carrots, diced bell peppers)

For the Tahini Dressing:

• 2 tablespoons tahini

• 1 tablespoon olive oil

• 1 tablespoon lemon juice

• 1 clove garlic, minced

• Salt and pepper to taste

• Water (for thinning, if necessary)

Instructions:

Cook Quinoa:

1. Rinse 1 cup of quinoa under cold water. Combine quinoa with 2 cups of water in a saucepan.

2. Bring to a boil, then reduce heat to low, cover, and simmer for 15 minutes or until the quinoa is cooked and water is absorbed.

3. Fluff quinoa with a fork and set aside.

Prepare Grilled Chicken or Chickpeas:

1. Grill chicken breast strips until fully cooked or use canned chickpeas, rinsed and drained.

Cook Mixed Vegetables:

1. Steam or sauté broccoli florets, sliced carrots, and diced bell peppers until tender-crisp.

Prepare Tahini Dressing:

1. In a small bowl, whisk together tahini, olive oil, lemon juice, minced garlic, salt, and pepper.

2. If the dressing is too thick, add water a tablespoon at a time until desired consistency is reached.

Assemble Quinoa Power Bowl:

1. In serving bowls, layer cooked quinoa as the base.

2. Top with grilled chicken or chickpeas.

3. Arrange the mixed vegetables on top.

4. Drizzle the Tahini Dressing over the bowl.

Garnish (Optional):

1. Garnish with fresh herbs like chopped parsley or a sprinkle of sesame seeds.

Nutritional Information (Per Serving):

• Calories: Approximately 400 kcal

• Protein: 20g (varies based on choice of protein)

• Fat: 15g

• Carbohydrates: 50g

• Fiber: 8g

• Sugar: 3g

Note:

• The Quinoa Power Bowl is a nutrient-dense meal combining whole grains, lean protein, and a variety of colorful vegetables.

• Quinoa provides complete protein and essential amino acids.

• The tahini dressing adds healthy fats and a rich, nutty flavor.

• This versatile bowl can be customized with your favorite vegetables and protein sources.

• It serves as a satisfying lunch or dinner option, promoting metabolic health through a well-rounded and flavorful combination of ingredients.

Mediterranean Salad Delight

Ingredients:

For the Salad:

• Mixed greens (spinach, arugula, and romaine), washed and chopped

• Cherry tomatoes, halved

• Cucumber, sliced

• Kalamata olives, pitted

• Feta cheese, crumbled

• Grilled shrimp or tofu (seasoned to taste)

For the Dressing:

• 3 tablespoons extra virgin olive oil

• 1 tablespoon balsamic vinegar

• 1 teaspoon Dijon mustard

• 1 clove garlic, minced

• Salt and pepper to taste

Instructions:

Prepare Salad:

1. Greens and Veggies:

o In a large bowl, combine the mixed greens, halved cherry tomatoes, sliced cucumber, Kalamata olives, and crumbled feta cheese.

2. Protein Choice:

o If using shrimp, ensure they are grilled until opaque and seasoned to taste.

o If using tofu, grill or pan-fry until golden and season to taste.

Make Dressing:

1. Whisk Dressing:

o In a small bowl, whisk together extra virgin olive oil, balsamic vinegar, Dijon mustard, minced garlic, salt, and pepper until well combined.

2. Adjust Seasoning:

o Taste the dressing and adjust salt and pepper according to your preference.

Assemble Salad:

1. Add Protein:

o Place the grilled shrimp or tofu on top of the salad.

2. Drizzle Dressing:

o Drizzle the prepared dressing over the entire salad.

3. Gently Toss:

o Gently toss the salad to coat the ingredients with the dressing evenly.

4. Garnish (Optional):

o Garnish with additional feta cheese and a sprinkle of fresh herbs like oregano or parsley.

Nutritional Information (Per Serving):

• Calories: Approximately 350 kcal

• Protein: 25g (varies based on choice of protein)

• Fat: 25g

• Carbohydrates: 15g

• Fiber: 5g

• Sugar: 5g

Note:

• The Mediterranean Salad Delight is a vibrant and flavorful dish that combines the freshness of vegetables with the richness of feta cheese and the protein of grilled shrimp or tofu.

• The dressing adds a zesty and tangy element to tie all the flavors together.

• This salad is not only delicious but also provides a variety of nutrients, supporting a balanced and metabolic-friendly diet.

• Enjoy it as a light lunch or dinner for a satisfying and healthful meal.

Wholesome Dinners to Wind Down:

Baked Salmon with Lemon Herb Quinoa

Ingredients:

• Salmon fillet

• 1 cup quinoa, uncooked

• 1 lemon, sliced

• Fresh herbs (dill or parsley), chopped

• Olive oil

• Salt and pepper to taste

Instructions:

Prepare Quinoa:

1. Rinse Quinoa:

o Rinse 1 cup of quinoa under cold water.

2. Cook Quinoa:

o Combine quinoa with 2 cups of water in a saucepan.

o Bring to a boil, then reduce heat to low, cover, and simmer for 15 minutes or until water is absorbed.

3. Fluff Quinoa:

o Fluff quinoa with a fork and set aside.

Prepare Salmon:

1. Preheat Oven:

o Preheat the oven to 375°F (190°C).

2. Season Salmon:

o Place the salmon fillet on a baking sheet lined with parchment paper.

o Drizzle with olive oil and season with salt, pepper, and chopped herbs.

3. Add Lemon Slices:

o Arrange lemon slices on top of the salmon.

4. Bake Salmon:

o Bake in the preheated oven for 15-20 minutes or until the salmon is cooked through and flakes easily with a fork.

Assemble Dish:

1. Flavor Quinoa:

o While the salmon is baking, add a squeeze of lemon juice and a drizzle of olive oil to the cooked quinoa.

o Mix in the chopped herbs.

2. Serve:

o Spoon a portion of lemon herb quinoa onto each plate.

3. Top with Salmon:

o Place a portion of the baked salmon on top of the quinoa.

4. Garnish (Optional):

o Garnish with additional chopped herbs and lemon slices.

Nutritional Information (Per Serving):

• Calories: Approximately 400 kcal

• Protein: 30g

• Fat: 20g

• Carbohydrates: 25g

• Fiber: 4g

• Sugar: 1g

Note:

• Baked Salmon with Lemon Herb Quinoa is a wholesome and protein-packed meal.

• Salmon provides omega-3 fatty acids and high-quality protein.

• Quinoa adds fiber and additional protein.

• The lemon and herbs contribute fresh and zesty flavors.

• This dish is not only delicious but also supports metabolic health through a balance of nutrients.

• Enjoy this nutrient-rich meal for a satisfying and nourishing dinner.

Stir-Fried Tofu with Rainbow Vegetables

Ingredients:

• 14 oz (400g) firm tofu, pressed and cubed

• 1 red bell pepper, thinly sliced

• 1 yellow bell pepper, thinly sliced

• 1 zucchini, thinly sliced

• 1 cup broccoli florets

• 2 tablespoons soy sauce

• 2 tablespoons vegetable oil

• 1 teaspoon sesame oil (optional)

• 1 tablespoon fresh ginger, minced

• 2 cloves garlic, minced

• Green onions for garnish (optional)

• Sesame seeds for garnish (optional)

• Cooked brown rice or quinoa (optional, for serving)

Instructions:

Prepare Tofu:

1. Press Tofu:

o Press the tofu between paper towels or using a tofu press to remove excess moisture. Cut into 1-inch cubes.

Stir-Fry:

1. Heat Pan:

o Heat vegetable oil in a wok or large pan over medium-high heat.

2. Sauté Tofu:

o Add cubed tofu to the hot pan and stir-fry until golden brown on all sides, about 5-7 minutes.

3. Add Vegetables:

o Add sliced bell peppers, zucchini, and broccoli florets to the pan. Stir-fry for an additional 5-7 minutes until the vegetables are tender-crisp.

4. Prepare Sauce:

o In a small bowl, mix soy sauce, and sesame oil (if using).

5. Combine Sauce:

o Pour the sauce over the tofu and vegetables. Toss everything together to ensure an even coating.

6. Add Aromatics:

o Add minced ginger and garlic to the pan. Stir-fry for an additional 2-3 minutes until fragrant.

7. Finish Cooking:

o Continue to stir-fry for an additional 2-3 minutes, allowing the flavors to meld and the sauce to thicken slightly.

8. Garnish and Serve:

o Garnish with chopped green onions and sesame seeds if desired.

Serve:

1. Optional Base:

o Serve the stir-fried tofu and vegetables over cooked brown rice or quinoa if desired.

Nutritional Information (Per Serving):

• Calories: Approximately 300 kcal

• Protein: 18g

• Fat: 20g

• Carbohydrates: 15g

• Fiber: 5g

• Sugar: 5g

Note:

• Stir-Fried Tofu with Rainbow Vegetables is a colorful and nutrient-packed dish that combines the protein of tofu with the vitamins and minerals of various vegetables.

• Pressing the tofu ensures a firmer texture and better absorption of flavors.

• Feel free to customize the vegetables based on personal preferences or seasonal availability.

• Serve over brown rice or quinoa for a complete and satisfying meal that supports metabolic health through a diverse array of plant-based nutrients.

Protein-Packed Omelet with Avocado

Ingredients:

• 3 large eggs

• 1/4 cup diced bell peppers (mix of colors)

• 2 tablespoons diced onions

• 1/4 cup cherry tomatoes, halved

• 2 tablespoons crumbled feta cheese

• 1/2 ripe avocado, sliced

• Salt and pepper to taste

• 1 tablespoon olive oil (for cooking)

Instructions:

Prepare Vegetables:

1. Dice Vegetables:

o Dice bell peppers, onions, and halve cherry tomatoes.

Whisk Eggs:

1. Whisk Eggs:

o In a bowl, crack the eggs and whisk them until well

combined.

o Season with a pinch of salt and pepper.

Preheat Pan:

1. Heat Olive Oil:

o Heat olive oil in a non-stick skillet over medium heat.

Sauté Vegetables:

1. Sauté Onions and Peppers:

o Add diced onions and bell peppers to the pan.

o Sauté until the vegetables are softened, about 2-3 minutes.

Add Eggs to the Pan:

1. Pour Whisked Eggs:

o Pour the whisked eggs over the sautéed vegetables in the pan.

Cook the Omelet:

1. Set Edges:

o Allow the eggs to set slightly at the edges.

2. Lift Edges:

o Gently lift the edges of the omelet with a spatula, allowing uncooked eggs to flow underneath.

Add Tomatoes and Feta:

1. Sprinkle Tomatoes and Feta:

o Sprinkle halved cherry tomatoes and crumbled feta cheese over one half of the omelet.

Fold and Serve:

1. Fold the Omelet:

o Once the eggs are mostly set but still slightly runny on top, fold the omelet in half using the spatula.

2. Cook Through:

o Continue cooking for an additional 1-2 minutes until the cheese melts, and the omelet is cooked through.

Plate and Garnish:

1. Transfer to a Plate:

o Carefully transfer the omelet to a plate.

2. Top with Avocado:

o Top the omelet with sliced avocado.

Season and Serve:

1. Season and Garnish:

o Season the omelet with additional salt and pepper if needed.

o Garnish with fresh herbs or a sprinkle of feta if desired.

Nutritional Information (Per Serving):

• Calories: Approximately 350 kcal

• Protein: 20g

• Fat: 25g

• Carbohydrates: 12g

• Fiber: 5g

• Sugar: 3g

Note:

• This Protein-Packed Omelet with Avocado is a balanced and satiating meal, providing a good source of protein, healthy fats, and essential nutrients.

• Bell peppers and tomatoes contribute vitamins C and A, while onions add flavor and additional nutrients.

• Feta cheese offers a tangy kick and a dose of calcium.

• Avocado adds creaminess and heart-healthy monounsaturated fats.

• This omelet is suitable for breakfast, brunch, or a quick and nutritious dinner, supporting your metabolic health with a delicious and satisfying combination of ingredients.

Quinoa Power Bowl

Ingredients:

For the Bowl:

• 1 cup quinoa, uncooked

• Grilled chicken breast strips or cooked chickpeas

• Mixed vegetables (broccoli florets, sliced carrots, diced bell peppers)

For the Tahini Dressing:

• 2 tablespoons tahini

• 1 tablespoon olive oil

• 1 tablespoon lemon juice

• 1 clove garlic, minced

• Salt and pepper to taste

• Water (for thinning, if necessary)

Instructions:

Cook Quinoa:

1. Rinse Quinoa:

o Rinse 1 cup of quinoa under cold water.

2. Cook Quinoa:

o Combine quinoa with 2 cups of water in a saucepan.

o Bring to a boil, then reduce heat to low, cover, and simmer for 15 minutes or until water is absorbed.

3. Fluff Quinoa:

o Fluff quinoa with a fork and set aside.

Prepare Grilled Chicken or Chickpeas:

1. Grill Chicken or Chickpeas:

o Grill chicken breast strips until fully cooked, or use canned chickpeas, rinsed and drained.

Cook Mixed Vegetables:

1. Steam or Sauté Vegetables:

o Steam or sauté broccoli florets, sliced carrots, and diced bell peppers until tender-crisp.

Prepare Tahini Dressing:

1. Whisk Dressing:

o In a small bowl, whisk together tahini, olive oil, lemon juice, minced garlic, salt, and pepper.

2. Adjust Seasoning:

o Taste the dressing and adjust salt and pepper according to your preference.

Assemble Quinoa Power Bowl:

1. Layer Quinoa:

o In serving bowls, layer cooked quinoa as the base.

2. Top with Protein:

o Top with grilled chicken or chickpeas.

3. Add Vegetables:

o Arrange the mixed vegetables on top.

4. Drizzle with Dressing:

o Drizzle the Tahini Dressing over the bowl.

Garnish (Optional):

1. Add Fresh Herbs:

o Garnish with fresh herbs like chopped parsley or a sprinkle of sesame seeds.

Nutritional Information (Per Serving):

• Calories: Approximately 400 kcal

• Protein: 20g (varies based on choice of protein)

• Fat: 15g

• Carbohydrates: 50g

• Fiber: 8g

• Sugar: 3g

Note:

• The Quinoa Power Bowl is a nutrient-dense meal combining whole grains, lean protein, and a variety of colorful vegetables.

• Quinoa provides complete protein and essential amino

acids.

• The tahini dressing adds healthy fats and a rich, nutty flavor.

• This versatile bowl can be customized with your favorite vegetables and protein sources.

• It serves as a satisfying lunch or dinner option, promoting metabolic health through a well-rounded and flavorful combination of ingredients.

Mediterranean Salad Delight

Ingredients:

For the Salad:

• Mixed greens (spinach, arugula, and romaine), washed and chopped

• Cherry tomatoes, halved

• Cucumber, sliced

• Kalamata olives, pitted

• Feta cheese, crumbled

• Grilled shrimp or tofu (seasoned to taste)

For the Dressing:

• 3 tablespoons extra virgin olive oil

• 1 tablespoon balsamic vinegar

• 1 teaspoon Dijon mustard

• 1 clove garlic, minced

• Salt and pepper to taste

Instructions:

Prepare Salad:

1. Greens and Veggies:

o In a large bowl, combine the mixed greens, halved cherry tomatoes, sliced cucumber, Kalamata olives, and crumbled feta cheese.

2. Protein Choice:

o If using shrimp, ensure they are grilled until opaque and seasoned to taste.

o If using tofu, grill or pan-fry until golden and season to taste.

Make Dressing:

1. Whisk Dressing:

o In a small bowl, whisk together extra virgin olive oil, balsamic vinegar, Dijon mustard, minced garlic, salt, and pepper until well combined.

2. Adjust Seasoning:

o Taste the dressing and adjust salt and pepper according to your preference.

Assemble Salad:

1. Add Protein:

o Place the grilled shrimp or tofu on top of the salad.

2. Drizzle Dressing:

o Drizzle the prepared dressing over the entire salad.

3. Gently Toss:

o Gently toss the salad to coat the ingredients with the dressing evenly.

4. Garnish (Optional):

o Garnish with additional feta cheese and a sprinkle of fresh herbs like oregano or parsley.

Nutritional Information (Per Serving):

• Calories: Approximately 350 kcal

• Protein: 25g (varies based on choice of protein)

• Fat: 25g

• Carbohydrates: 15g

• Fiber: 5g

• Sugar: 5g

Note:

• The Mediterranean Salad Delight is a vibrant and flavorful dish that combines the freshness of vegetables with the richness of feta cheese and the protein of grilled shrimp or tofu.

• The dressing adds a zesty and tangy element to tie all the flavors together.

• This salad is not only delicious but also provides a variety of nutrients, supporting a balanced and metabolic-friendly diet.

• Enjoy it as a light lunch or dinner for a satisfying and healthful meal.

.

Sweet Treats to Satisfy Cravings:

Dark Chocolate Berry Delight

Ingredients:

• Dark chocolate squares (70% cocoa or higher)

• Mixed berries (strawberries, blueberries, raspberries)

Instructions:

Prepare Berries:

1. Wash and Dry Berries:

o Wash the berries thoroughly and pat them dry with a paper towel.

Melt Dark Chocolate:

1. Double Boiler Method:

o Break the dark chocolate squares into small pieces and place them in a heatproof bowl.

o Use a double boiler to melt the chocolate, stirring constantly until smooth.

o Alternatively, melt the chocolate in short bursts in the microwave, stirring after each interval.

Dip Berries:

1. Dip Berries in Chocolate:

o Hold each berry by its stem and dip it into the melted dark chocolate, ensuring it's well-coated.

2. Place on Parchment:

o Place the chocolate-coated berries on a parchment paper-lined tray or plate.

3. Repeat for All Berries:

o Repeat the dipping process for each berry.

Chill:

1. Refrigerate:

o Place the tray of chocolate-covered berries in the refrigerator for at least 30 minutes or until the chocolate hardens.

Serve:

1. Arrange on a Plate:

o Once the chocolate has set, arrange the Dark Chocolate Berry Delights on a serving plate.

Nutritional Information (Per Serving):

• Calories: Approximately 150 kcal (varies based on the amount of chocolate and berries)

• Fat: 10g

• Carbohydrates: 15g

• Protein: 2g

• Fiber: 5g

• Sugar: 8g

Note:

• Dark Chocolate Berry Delight is a simple and indulgent treat that combines the richness of dark chocolate with the freshness of mixed berries.

• Dark chocolate contains antioxidants and may offer various health benefits in moderation.

• Berries contribute vitamins, minerals, and fiber, adding a nutritious element to this delightful dessert.

• Enjoy these treats in moderation as a satisfying and metabolism-friendly dessert option.

Greek Yogurt Parfait

Ingredients:

• Greek yogurt

• Granola

• Honey

• Mixed fruits (kiwi, mango, berries)

Instructions:

Prepare Ingredients:

1. Dice Fruits:

o Dice the kiwi and mango into small, bite-sized pieces.

Assemble Parfait:

1. Layer Greek Yogurt:

o Begin by spooning a layer of Greek yogurt into the bottom of a glass or a bowl.

2. Add Granola:

o Sprinkle a layer of granola over the Greek yogurt. Choose a granola that is low in added sugars for a healthier option.

3. Drizzle Honey:

o Drizzle a small amount of honey over the granola for sweetness. Adjust the amount based on your taste preferences.

4. Add Mixed Fruits:

o Add a layer of mixed fruits, including diced kiwi, mango,

and berries.

5. Repeat Layers:

o Repeat the layers until you reach the top of the glass or bowl, finishing with a final layer of mixed fruits on top.

Nutritional Information (Per Serving):

• Calories: Approximately 300 kcal (varies based on portion sizes and ingredients)

• Protein: 15g

• Fat: 8g

• Carbohydrates: 45g

• Fiber: 6g

• Sugar: 20g

Note:

• The Greek Yogurt Parfait is a delicious and nutrient-packed snack or breakfast option that combines the creaminess of Greek yogurt with the crunch of granola and the natural sweetness of fruits.

• Greek yogurt provides protein and probiotics, granola offers fiber and energy, and mixed fruits contribute vitamins and antioxidants.

• Drizzling honey adds a touch of sweetness without overpowering the natural flavors.

• Customize the parfait with your favorite fruits and granola flavors for a metabolism-friendly and satisfying treat.

Baked Salmon with Lemon Herb Quinoa

Ingredients:

• Salmon fillet

• Quinoa

• Lemon

• Fresh herbs (such as dill or parsley)

• Olive oil

• Salt and pepper to taste

Instructions:

Prepare Salmon:

1. Preheat Oven:

o Preheat the oven to 375°F (190°C).

2. Season Salmon:

o Place the salmon fillet on a baking sheet lined with parchment paper.

o Drizzle olive oil over the salmon and season with salt, pepper, and fresh herbs.

3. Bake Salmon:

o Bake the salmon in the preheated oven for 15-20 minutes or until the salmon is cooked through and flakes easily with a fork.

Prepare Quinoa:

1. Rinse Quinoa:

o Rinse 1 cup of quinoa under cold water.

2. Cook Quinoa:

o Combine quinoa with 2 cups of water in a saucepan.

o Bring to a boil, then reduce heat to low, cover, and simmer for 15 minutes or until water is absorbed.

3. Fluff Quinoa:

o Fluff quinoa with a fork and add a squeeze of lemon juice, fresh herbs, salt, and pepper to taste.

Serve:

1. Plate Quinoa:

o Spoon a portion of lemon herb quinoa onto each plate.

2. Top with Salmon:

o Place a serving of baked salmon on top of the quinoa.

3. Garnish with Lemon:

o Garnish the dish with lemon slices and additional fresh herbs for a burst of flavor.

Nutritional Information (Per Serving):

• Calories: Approximately 400 kcal (varies based on portion sizes and ingredients)

• Protein: 30g

• Fat: 20g

• Carbohydrates: 25g

• Fiber: 4g

• Sugar: 1g

Note:

• Baked Salmon with Lemon Herb Quinoa is a well-balanced and nutritious meal that provides omega-3 fatty acids from salmon, protein from quinoa, and a refreshing twist from lemon and herbs.

• This dish is rich in healthy fats, vitamins, and minerals, supporting a metabolism-friendly and health-conscious diet.

• Adjust the quantities based on your dietary needs and preferences, and enjoy this flavorful and satisfying meal as part of your metabolic confusion diet.

Stir-Fried Tofu with Rainbow Vegetables

Ingredients:

• Tofu, extra firm, pressed and cubed

• Bell peppers (a mix of colors), sliced

• Zucchini, sliced

• Broccoli florets

• Soy sauce (low-sodium)

• Sesame oil

• Garlic, minced

• Ginger, grated

• Olive oil for cooking

• Green onions, chopped (for garnish)

• Sesame seeds (optional, for garnish)

Instructions:

Prepare Tofu:

1. Press Tofu:

o Press the extra firm tofu to remove excess water. Place the tofu between paper towels and press with a heavy object for at least 15-20 minutes.

2. Cube Tofu:

o Cut the pressed tofu into cubes.

Stir-Fry Tofu:

1. Sear Tofu:

o Heat olive oil in a wok or large skillet over medium-high heat.

o Add tofu cubes and sear until golden brown on all sides.

2. Remove Tofu:

o Once browned, remove tofu from the wok and set aside.

Stir-Fry Vegetables:

1. Sauté Aromatics:

o In the same wok, add a bit more olive oil if needed. Sauté minced garlic and grated ginger until fragrant.

2. Add Vegetables:

o Add bell peppers, zucchini, and broccoli to the wok.

o Stir-fry until the vegetables are tender-crisp but still vibrant.

Combine Tofu and Vegetables:

1. Reintroduce Tofu:

o Return the seared tofu to the wok with the sautéed

vegetables.

2. Soy Sauce:

o Pour in low-sodium soy sauce and a splash of sesame oil.

o Toss everything together until well-coated.

3. Finish Cooking:

o Stir-fry for an additional 2-3 minutes, allowing the flavors to meld.

Garnish and Serve:

1. Garnish:

o Garnish the stir-fry with chopped green onions and sesame seeds if desired.

Nutritional Information (Per Serving):

• Calories: Approximately 300 kcal (varies based on portion sizes and ingredients)

• Protein: 15g

• Fat: 20g

• Carbohydrates: 15g

• Fiber: 5g

• Sugar: 5g

Note:

• Stir-Fried Tofu with Rainbow Vegetables is a colorful and flavorful dish that provides plant-based protein and a variety of vitamins and minerals.

• Tofu serves as a protein source, while the rainbow of vegetables adds a mix of nutrients.

• The stir-fry is seasoned with soy sauce and sesame oil for a savory and umami flavor profile.

• Enjoy this dish on its own or serve it over brown rice or quinoa for a complete and metabolism-friendly meal.

Protein-Packed Omelet with Avocado

Ingredients:

• Eggs

• Diced bell peppers (a mix of colors)

• Onions, finely chopped

• Cherry tomatoes, halved

• Feta cheese, crumbled

• Avocado, sliced

• Olive oil or cooking spray

• Salt and pepper to taste

• Fresh herbs (such as parsley or chives), chopped (optional, for garnish)

Instructions:

Prepare Vegetables:

1. Chop Ingredients:

o Dice bell peppers, finely chop onions, and halve cherry tomatoes. Crumble the feta cheese.

Cook Vegetables:

1. Sauté Vegetables:

o Heat olive oil or cooking spray in a non-stick skillet over medium heat.

o Sauté onions and bell peppers until softened and slightly caramelized.

2. Add Tomatoes:

o Add cherry tomatoes to the skillet and cook briefly until they just start to soften.

3. Remove from Heat:

o Transfer the sautéed vegetables to a plate and set aside.

Prepare Eggs:

1. Whisk Eggs:

o In a bowl, whisk the eggs until well combined. Season with salt and pepper.

2. Cook Eggs:

o Heat the skillet again over medium heat. Add a bit more oil or cooking spray if needed.

o Pour the whisked eggs into the skillet.

3. Create Omelet:

o As the edges of the eggs start to set, gently lift them with a spatula, allowing the uncooked eggs to flow underneath.

4. Add Vegetables and Feta:

o Once the eggs are mostly set but still slightly runny on top, add the sautéed vegetables and crumbled feta cheese on one half of the omelet.

5. Fold and Finish Cooking:

o Carefully fold the other half of the omelet over the filling.

o Continue cooking for another minute or until the eggs are fully set and the cheese is melted.

Serve:

1. Plate Omelet:

o Slide the protein-packed omelet onto a plate.

2. Top with Avocado:

o Top the omelet with sliced avocado.

3. Garnish:

o Garnish with fresh herbs if desired.

Nutritional Information (Per Serving):

• Calories: Approximately 350 kcal (varies based on portion sizes and ingredients)

• Protein: 20g

• Fat: 25g

• Carbohydrates: 10g

• Fiber: 4g

• Sugar: 5g

Note:

• The Protein-Packed Omelet with Avocado is a nutritious and satisfying breakfast option rich in protein, healthy fats, and vegetables.

• Customize the omelet with your favorite vegetables and herbs to suit your taste preferences.

• The addition of avocado provides creamy texture and additional healthy fats.

• Enjoy this protein-packed meal to kickstart your day with a metabolism-friendly and delicious breakfast.

Hydration with a Twist:

Infused Water Elixir

Ingredients:

• Cucumber slices

• Mint leaves

• Lemon slices

Instructions:

Prepare Ingredients:

1. Slice Cucumber:

o Wash and slice a cucumber into thin rounds.

2. Prepare mint leaves:

o Wash a handful of fresh mint leaves, pat them dry, and gently bruise them to release their flavours.

3. Slice Lemon:

o Slice a lemon into thin rounds.

Assemble infused water:

1. Combine Ingredients:

o In a large pitcher, combine the cucumber slices, mint leaves, and lemon slices.

2. Add Water:

o Fill the pitcher with cold, filtered water. Use

approximately 1.5 to 2 litres, depending on the size of your pitcher.

3. Refrigerate:

o Place the pitcher in the refrigerator and let the ingredients infuse for at least 2-4 hours or overnight for a more intense flavour.

Serve:

1. Pour and enjoy:

o Pour the infused water into glasses, allowing some cucumber, mint, and lemon slices to be served in each glass.

2. Refresh:

o Refresh the water in the pitcher as needed. The infused water can last in the refrigerator for up to 24 hours.

Nutritional Information (Per Serving):

• Calories: approximately 0 kcal (infused water is low in calories).

• There are no significant amounts of macronutrients, as this is primarily water with infused flavours.

Note:

• The Infused Water Elixir is a refreshing and hydrating drink that adds a burst of natural flavours without added sugars or calories.

• Cucumber provides a subtle freshness, mint adds a hint of coolness, and lemon contributes a zesty kick.

• This elixir not only keeps you hydrated but also encourages water consumption with its appealing taste.

• Enjoy this drink as a healthy alternative to sugary

beverages and stay refreshed throughout the day.

.

Dark Chocolate Berry Delight

Ingredients:

• Dark chocolate squares (70% cocoa or higher)

• Mixed berries (strawberries, blueberries, raspberries)

Instructions:

Prepare Berries:

1. Wash and Dry Berries:

o Wash the berries thoroughly and pat them dry with a paper towel.

Melt dark chocolate:

1. Double Boiler Method:

o Break the dark chocolate squares into small pieces and place them in a heatproof bowl.

o Use a double boiler to melt the chocolate, stirring constantly until smooth.

o Alternatively, melt the chocolate in short bursts in the microwave, stirring after each interval.

Dip Berries:

1. Dip Berries in Chocolate:

o Hold each berry by its stem and dip it into the melted dark chocolate, ensuring it's well coated.

2. Place on Parchment:

o Place the chocolate-coated berries on a parchment-paper-lined tray or plate.

3. Repeat for all berries:

o Repeat the dipping process for each berry.

Chill:

1. Refrigerate:

o Place the tray of chocolate-covered berries in the refrigerator for at least 30 minutes, or until the chocolate hardens.

Serve:

1. Arrange on a plate:

o Once the chocolate has set, arrange the Dark Chocolate Berry Delights on a serving plate.

Nutritional Information (Per Serving):

• Calories: approximately 150 kcal (varies based on the amount of chocolate and berries).

• Fat: 10g

• Carbohydrates: 15g

• Protein: 2g

• Fibre: 5g

• Sugar: 8g

Note:

• Dark Chocolate Berry Delight is a simple and indulgent treat that combines the richness of dark chocolate with the freshness of mixed berries.

• Dark chocolate contains antioxidants and may offer various health benefits in moderation.

• Berries contribute vitamins, minerals, and fibre, adding a nutritious element to this delightful dessert.

• Enjoy these treats in moderation as a satisfying and metabolism-friendly dessert option.

Greek Yoghurt Parfait

Ingredients:

• Greek yoghurt

• Granola

• Honey

• Mixed fruits (kiwi, mango, berries)

Instructions:

Prepare Ingredients:

1. Dice Fruits:

o Dice the kiwi and mango into small, bite-sized pieces. Wash the berries if needed.

2. Layer Greek Yoghurt:

o Begin by spooning a layer of Greek yoghurt into the bottom of a glass or a bowl.

3. Add Granola:

o Sprinkle a layer of granola over the Greek yogurt. Choose a granola that is low in added sugars for a healthier option.

4. Drizzle Honey:

o Drizzle a small amount of honey over the granola for sweetness. Adjust the amount based on your taste preferences.

5. Add mixed fruits:

o Add a layer of mixed fruits, including diced kiwi, mango, and berries.

6. Repeat Layers:

o Repeat the layers until you reach the top of the glass or bowl, finishing with a final layer of mixed fruits on top.

Serve:

1. Garnish:

o Optionally, garnish the top with a few whole berries or a slice of kiwi for an attractive presentation.

Nutritional Information (Per Serving):

• Calories: approximately 300 kcal (varies based on portion sizes and ingredients).

• Protein: 15g

• Fat: 8g

• Carbohydrates: 45g

• Fibre: 6g

• Sugar: 20g

Note:

• The Greek Yoghurt Parfait is a delicious and nutrient-packed snack or breakfast option that combines the creaminess of Greek yoghurt with the crunch of granola and the natural sweetness of fruits.

• Greek yoghurt provides protein and probiotics; granola offers fibre and energy; and mixed fruits contribute vitamins and antioxidants.

• Drizzling honey adds a touch of sweetness without

overpowering the natural flavours.

• Customise the parfait with your favourite fruits and granola flavours for a metabolism-friendly and delightful treat.

Baked Salmon with Lemon Herb Quinoa

Ingredients:

• Salmon fillet

• Quinoa

• Lemon

• Fresh herbs (such as dill or parsley)

• Olive oil

• Salt and pepper to taste

Instructions:

Prepare Salmon:

1. Preheat Oven:

o Preheat the oven to 375°F (190°C).

2. Season Salmon:

o Place the salmon fillet on a baking sheet lined with parchment paper.

o Drizzle olive oil over the salmon and season with salt, pepper, and fresh herbs.

3. Bake Salmon:

o Bake the salmon in the preheated oven for 15-20 minutes

or until the salmon is cooked through and flakes easily with a fork.

Prepare Quinoa:

1. Rinse Quinoa:

o Rinse 1 cup of quinoa in cold water.

2. Cook Quinoa:

o Combine quinoa with 2 cups of water in a saucepan.

o Bring to a boil, then reduce heat to low, cover, and simmer for 15 minutes or until water is absorbed.

3. Fluff Quinoa:

o Fluff quinoa with a fork and add a squeeze of lemon juice, fresh herbs, salt, and pepper to taste.

Serve:

1. Plate Quinoa:

o Spoon a portion of lemon-herb quinoa onto each plate.

2. Top with salmon:

o Place a serving of baked salmon on top of the quinoa.

3. Garnish with lemon.

o Garnish the dish with lemon slices and additional fresh herbs for a burst of flavour.

Nutritional Information (Per Serving):

• Calories: approximately 400 kcal (varies based on portion sizes and ingredients).

• Protein: 30g

• Fat: 20g

• Carbohydrates: 25g

• Fibre: 4g

• Sugar: 1g

Note:

• Baked Salmon with Lemon Herb Quinoa is a well-balanced and nutritious meal that provides omega-3 fatty acids from salmon, protein from quinoa, and a refreshing twist from lemon and herbs.

• This dish is rich in healthy fats, vitamins, and minerals, supporting a metabolism-friendly and health-conscious diet.

• Adjust the quantities based on your dietary needs and preferences, and enjoy this flavorful and satisfying meal as part of your metabolic confusion diet.

◆ ◆ ◆

CONCLUSION

As we draw the final curtain on this exploration of the Metabolic Confusion Diet, it's not just an end but a commencement—a commencement of a lifelong journey towards metabolic wellness, balance, and sustainable health. The pages of this book have unfolded the principles, recipes, and insights that form the foundation of a lifestyle that transcends the limitations of conventional diets.

In the realm of metabolic confusion, we've discovered the power of variability—variability in caloric intake, macronutrient ratios, and lifestyle practices. It's a paradigm shift that transcends the rigidity of one-size-fits-all approaches, recognising the uniqueness of each individual's metabolic fingerprint. The journey of metabolic confusion is not about restriction; it's about liberation—a liberation from the shackles of unsustainable diets and a celebration of the body's innate ability to adapt, thrive, and find balance.

As you embark on this journey, armed with knowledge and a palette of flavorful recipes, remember that metabolic wellness is not a destination but a continuous process of learning and refinement. It's about embracing the ebb and flow of life and recognising that health is not an isolated pursuit but a harmonious integration of mindful nutrition, physical activity, and self-awareness.

In the world of metabolic confusion, there are no failures —only lessons. Each experiment, every recipe, and all the small victories contribute to a mosaic of well-being. Listen to your body, honour its signals, and relish the joy of nourishing it with a rich tapestry of nutrient-dense foods.

The Metabolic Confusion Diet is not a rigid rulebook but a flexible guide, allowing you to tailor its principles to your unique preferences and circumstances. It's a call to mindfulness—a call to savour the journey, savour the flavours, and savour the moments that contribute to a life of vitality.

So, as you close this chapter and step into the realm of metabolic well-being, remember that you are the author of your health story. May your journey be filled with vibrant, nourishing meals, invigorating physical activity, and a profound sense of well-being. Here's to a life where metabolic confusion becomes metabolic clarity—a clarity that stems from balance, adaptation, and the unwavering belief that your body is a resilient, dynamic masterpiece.

Cheers to your journey of metabolic wellness!